RENAL DIET

COOKBOOK

FOR NEWLY DIAGNOSED

1000 DAY RECIPES

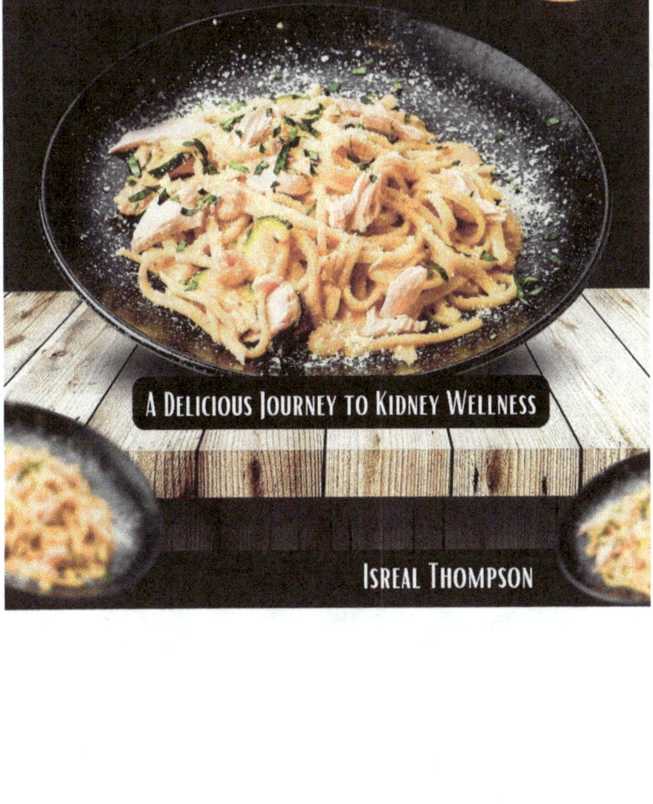

A Delicious Journey to Kidney Wellness

ISREAL THOMPSON

Renal diet

Cookbook

For newly diagnosed

Ignite your journey to Kidney health

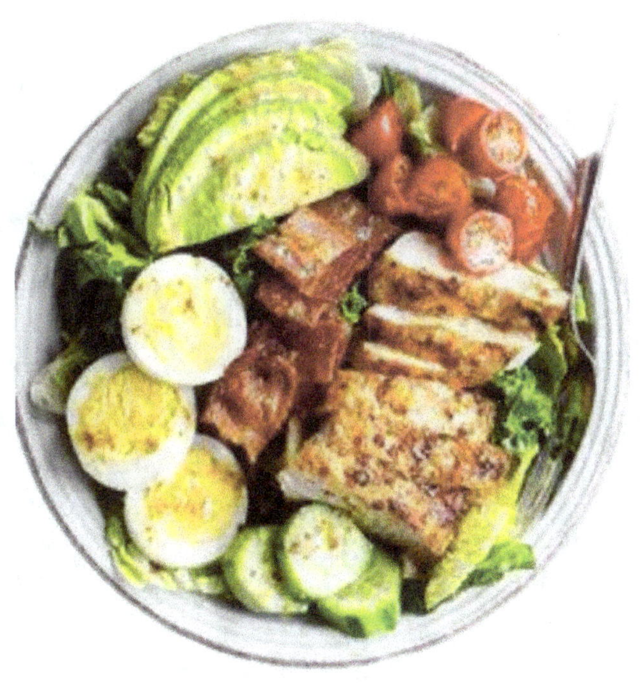

TABLE OF CONTENTS

Chapter 1: Introduction   **5**

Understanding Renal Diets   8

Tips for Newly Diagnosed Males   12

Basics of Renal Nutrition   16

Key Nutrients for Kidney Health   20

Breakfast Recipes   24

Cinnamon Oatmeal with Fresh Berries   27

Lunch and Dinner Entrees   30

Grilled Lemon Herb Chicken   33

Salmon with Dill Sauce   35

Lentil and Vegetable Stew   37

Snacks and Appetizers   39

Avocado and Tomato Salsa   42

Hummus with Crudites   44

Roasted Chickpeas   46

Chapter 2: Desserts   **48**

Berry Parfait with Greek Yogurt   50

Baked Apple with Cinnamon   52

Beverages   54

Hydration Tips for Kidney Health   56

Herbal Tea Infusions   59

Fruit-Infused Water Recipes   62

Conclusion   **64**

Chapter 1: Introduction

Welcome to "Renew: Nourishing Your Kidneys," a culinary journey designed exclusively for the newly diagnosed gentlemen seeking a harmonious fusion of flavor and kidney-friendly nourishment. Embarking on a renal diet doesn't mean bidding farewell to culinary delight; it's an invitation to discover a world of vibrant, wholesome, and utterly delectable recipes tailored to support your kidney health.

In these pages, you'll find more than just a collection of recipes; you'll find a compass guiding you through the transformative power of food. As you navigate this newly diagnosed terrain, "Renew" offers a compass, turning every meal into a step towards renewed well-being. From the sizzle of savory entrees to the sweetness of guilt-free desserts, we've crafted a symphony of flavors that not only caters to your dietary needs but celebrates the pleasure of eating.

Our culinary adventure begins with an understanding of renal nutrition, unraveling the mystery behind the choices we make to fuel our bodies. We delve into the art of balancing key nutrients, unlocking the secrets to maintaining optimal kidney function without compromising on taste. "Renew" is not just a cookbook; it's a companion, guiding you through the process of creating nourishing, kidney-friendly meals that invigorate the senses and nurture your well-being.

Prepare to embark on a gastronomic odyssey, where each recipe is a chapter in the story of your renewed health. Whether you're savoring a hearty breakfast, relishing a flavorsome dinner, or indulging in a guilt-free dessert, "Renew" is your passport to a world where taste and wellness coexist.

Embrace the journey, savor the flavors, and rediscover the joy of nourishing your kidneys—one delicious recipe at a time.

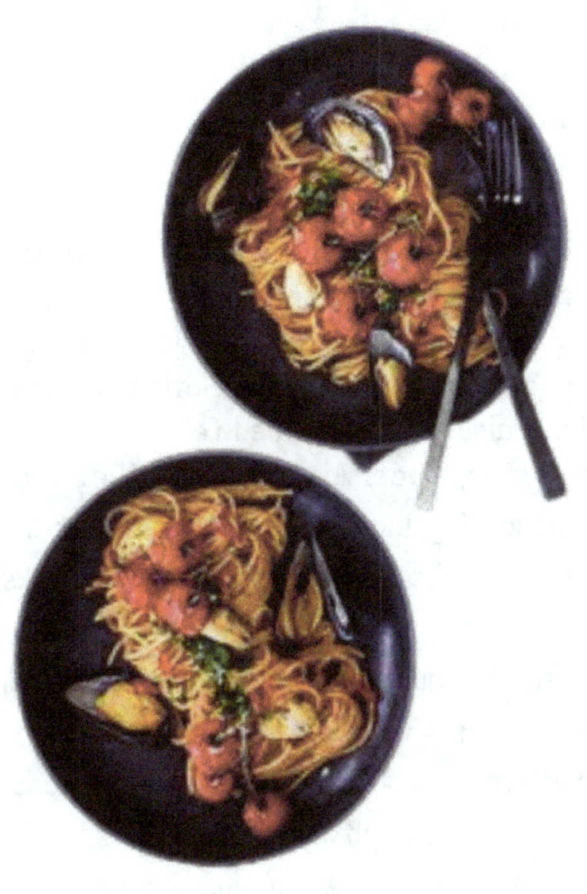

Understanding Renal Diets

Once upon a time in the vibrant town of Flavortopia, lived a curious soul named Alex. Alex, a recently diagnosed gentleman, embarked on a quest to unravel the secrets of renal diets—a journey that would not only redefine his relationship with food but also transform his life.

As the story goes, Alex's journey began at the enchanting Library of Nutrition, where ancient scrolls and modern cookbooks whispered tales of the delicate balance required to nurture kidney health. With each turn of the page, he discovered that renal diets weren't just about restrictions; they were a symphony of nutrients, each playing a vital role in maintaining the well-being of his precious kidneys.

Guided by a wise nutritionist named Chef Harmony, Alex learned that understanding renal diets was akin to composing a melody. The notes of potassium and phosphorus danced with proteins and fibers, creating a harmonious tune that resonated through every meal. Chef Harmony emphasized that the key to this culinary symphony lay in balance—a magical equilibrium that would allow Alex to savor the flavors of life while supporting his kidney health.

In the bustling market of Flavortopia, Alex's next adventure unfolded. Armed with a basket and Chef Harmony's guidance, he navigated the stalls like a culinary explorer. Together, they selected vibrant fruits, crisp vegetables, and lean proteins—ingredients that would become the building blocks of his kidney-friendly culinary creations.

The journey took an unexpected turn when they stumbled upon the Spice Bazaar, a magical place where the scents of cinnamon, cumin, and turmeric filled the air.

Chef Harmony revealed the secret alchemy of flavors, showing Alex how herbs and spices could transform his meals into a sensory delight without compromising on health.

Back in Alex's kitchen, the real magic happened. With Chef Harmony's wisdom, he experimented with recipes that tickled his taste buds and nourished his kidneys. From zesty breakfast burritos to succulent herb-infused chicken, each dish was a testament to the newfound understanding that health and flavor could coexist in perfect harmony.

As Alex savored the fruits of his culinary adventure, he realized that understanding renal diets wasn't just a dietary regimen; it was a tale of empowerment. He had become the hero of his own story, mastering the art of crafting meals that not only supported his kidney health but also brought joy to his palate.

And so, in the town of Flavortopia, the legend of Alex, the kidney-friendly chef, was born—a tale of understanding renal diets that echoed through the cobblestone streets, inspiring others to embark on their own flavorful adventures. For in every bite, there was harmony, and in every meal, a symphony of well-being played on, reminding all that the magic of understanding renal diets was within reach, waiting to be embraced. B. Importance of Nutrition for Kidney Health

Tips for Newly Diagnosed Males

Congratulations, gentlemen, on embarking on a journey towards renewed health! Being newly diagnosed brings its set of challenges, but fear not, for we have compiled a treasure trove of simple yet impactful tips to guide you through this new chapter.

1. Embrace Education

Knowledge is your greatest ally. Take the time to understand your diagnosis and learn about the basics of kidney health. Familiarize yourself with the concept of renal diets, and don't hesitate to ask your healthcare team any questions that arise.

2. Team Up with a Nutrition Sidekick

Meet your nutrition superhero—your friendly dietitian. Partnering with a nutrition expert can make crafting kidney-friendly meals a breeze. They'll help you navigate the culinary landscape, ensuring your diet supports your health goals without sacrificing taste.

3. Sip, Sip, Hooray

Hydration is key to kidney health. Make water your trusty sidekick and sip it throughout the day. It's a simple yet effective way to support your kidneys on their journey to wellness.

4. Portion Control Prowess

Master the art of portion control—it's your secret weapon. Keeping portions in check helps regulate nutrient intake without overwhelming your kidneys. Think of it as a mindful approach to enjoying your favorite foods.

5. Spice It Up

Elevate your meals with herbs and spices. They add a burst of flavor without the need for excess salt or other seasonings that might not be kidney-friendly.

Discover the magic of culinary herbs—your taste buds will thank you!

6. Make Friends with Fiber

Fiber is your digestive ally. Incorporate fiber-rich foods like fruits, vegetables, and whole grains into your diet. They not only contribute to overall well-being but also play a supportive role in kidney health.

7. Exercise – Your Secret Weapon

Engage in regular physical activity. It doesn't have to be a marathon; a simple daily stroll or activities you enjoy can do wonders. Exercise promotes overall health, which is a win-win for you and your kidneys.

8. Prioritize Protein

Opt for high-quality, lean proteins. They provide the essential amino acids your body needs without overloading your kidneys. Explore sources like poultry, fish, and plant-based proteins to keep your meals exciting.

9. Connect with Supportive Souls

You're not alone on this journey. Connect with others who share similar experiences, whether it's through support groups, online forums, or talking to friends and family. Sharing stories and advice can be a source of strength and inspiration.

10. Celebrate Small Wins

Finally, celebrate your victories, no matter how small. Each positive step you take towards a kidney-friendly lifestyle is a triumph. Remember, this journey is about progress, not perfection.

Armed with these simple yet impactful tips, gentlemen, you're ready to navigate the path to renewed health with confidence and a dash of flair. Here's to embracing the new normal and savoring every step of the journey!

Basics of Renal Nutrition

Embarking on a journey to understand renal nutrition? Fear not! Let's unravel the mysteries together and make kidney-friendly eating a breeze with these simple and captivating basics.

1. Hydration Elation

Water is your kidney's best friend. Stay hydrated by sipping water throughout the day. It's not just a drink; it's a hydrating high-five for your kidneys.

2. The Potassium Puzzle

Picture potassium as a friendly puzzle piece in your diet. While it's essential, too much can be a challenge for your kidneys. Embrace low-potassium heroes like apples, berries, and cabbage to keep the puzzle complete.

3. Phosphorus—The Stealthy Sidekick

Phosphorus is like a stealthy sidekick, hiding in unexpected places. Keep an eye on dairy, nuts, and processed foods, and opt for low-phosphorus alternatives to keep your kidneys happy.

4. The Protein Balance Beam

Protein is your ally, but balance is key. Opt for lean proteins like chicken, fish, and eggs. It's a balancing act that supports muscle health without overwhelming your kidneys.

5. Sodium Sensei

Meet Sodium Sensei, your guide to a low-sodium lifestyle. Dial down the salt and explore flavorful alternatives like herbs and spices. Your taste buds won't miss the extra sodium, and your kidneys will thank you.

6. Fiber: The Digestive Cheerleader

Fiber is your digestive cheerleader. Load up on fruits, veggies, and whole grains to keep things moving smoothly. It's a simple trick for happy tummies and content kidneys.

7. Portion Control Prowess

Master the art of portion control—it's like a superhero cape for your meals. Enjoy your favorite foods in moderation, ensuring a delightful dining experience without overwhelming your kidneys.

8. Mindful Meal Planning

Crafting kidney-friendly meals is like planning a culinary adventure. Mix and match nutrient-rich foods, experiment with new recipes, and discover the joy of nourishing your body while tantalizing your taste buds.

9. Culinary Creativity with Herbs and Spices

Spice up your meals with a dash of creativity. Herbs and spices are the artists in your culinary palette, adding flair without extra sodium.

Let your taste buds dance to the melody of flavorful, kidney-friendly dishes.

10. Personalized Plate Pleasure

Remember, renal nutrition is not a one-size-fits-all affair. Tailor your plate to your preferences and health needs. It's about creating a personalized, delicious symphony that suits your unique taste and nourishes your kidneys.

And there you have it—renal nutrition demystified and made simple. Armed with these basics, you're ready to embark on a flavorful journey that supports your kidney health with every delicious bite. Here's to happy, healthy eating!A. Overview of Renal Diet

Key Nutrients for Kidney Health

Embarking on a journey to nurture your kidneys? Let's navigate the nutrient landscape together and discover the key players that keep your kidneys smiling.

1. Water Wonders

Meet the hydration heroes! Water is not just a thirst quencher; it's a vital nutrient that flushes toxins, regulates temperature, and supports your kidneys in their daily work. Sip, sip, hooray for the elixir of life!

2. Potassium Power

Picture potassium as the powerhouse nutrient for your kidneys. Found in bananas, oranges, and sweet potatoes, it helps maintain fluid balance and keeps your heartbeat in check. Embrace the potassium power for a well-rounded diet.

3. Phosphorus—Balancing Act

Say hello to phosphorus, a nutrient that plays a balancing act in bone health. While it's essential, too much can be a challenge for your kidneys. Keep phosphorus in check by choosing wisely—nuts, dairy, and processed foods in moderation.

4. Protein Pal

Protein is your pal, supporting muscle health and keeping you energized. Opt for lean sources like chicken, fish, and eggs, maintaining a delicate balance that supports your kidneys without overwhelming them.

5. Sodium Smarts

Sodium, a sneaky character, hides in many foods. Practice sodium smarts by reducing salt and exploring flavorful alternatives. Your taste buds won't miss the extra salt, and your kidneys will appreciate the reduced workload.

6. Fiber Friends

Fiber, your digestive sidekick! Found in fruits, veggies, and whole grains, fiber keeps things moving smoothly. It's a friend to your digestive system and a key nutrient for overall well-being.

7. Iron Infusion

Iron, a nutrient superhero, plays a role in oxygen transport. Incorporate iron-rich foods like spinach, beans, and lean meats into your diet for a nutrient infusion that supports your overall health.

8. Calcium Companion

Calcium, the companion nutrient for strong bones and teeth. Milk, yogurt, and leafy greens are calcium-rich options that contribute to bone health without causing a calcium overload for your kidneys.

9. Vitamin D Dance

Join the vitamin D dance for strong bones and a vibrant immune system. Soak up some sunshine and include vitamin D-rich foods like fatty fish and fortified dairy products in your diet.

10. Magnesium Magic

Magnesium, the magic mineral, contributes to muscle and nerve function. Find it in nuts, seeds, and leafy greens to add a touch of magnesium magic to your nutrient mix.

Navigating the nutrient landscape is a journey of nourishment and care. With these key nutrients as your compass, you're equipped to cultivate a diet that not only tantalizes your taste buds but also supports the health and happiness of your kidneys. Here's to nutrient nurturing and a vibrant, kidney-friendly journey ahead!C. Portion Control and Meal Planning

Breakfast Recipes

Rise and shine, fellow kitchen adventurers! Let's kickstart your day with a burst of flavor and kidney-friendly goodness. These breakfast recipes are not only simple but also a delightful celebration of mornings.

1. Low-Potassium Breakfast Burrito

<u>Ingredients</u>

- 2 large eggs
- 1/4 cup diced bell peppers
- 1/4 cup diced tomatoes
-2 tablespoons shredded low-potassium cheese
- 1 whole wheat tortilla

<u>Preparation</u>:

1. Whisk eggs and cook with bell peppers and tomatoes until scrambled.

2. Sprinkle cheese on top and spoon the mixture onto a warm tortilla.

3. Roll it up, and your savory breakfast burrito is ready to savor!

2. Cinnamon Oatmeal with Fresh Berries

<u>Ingredients</u>:

- 1/2 cup old-fashioned oats

- 1 cup water or low-potassium milk

- 1/2 teaspoon ground cinnamon

- 1/4 cup fresh berries (blueberries, strawberries)

<u>Preparation</u>:

1. Cook oats with water or milk and stir in cinnamon.

2. Top with fresh berries, and let the warm aroma of cinnamon embrace your morning.

3. Egg White Vegetable Omelet:

<u>Ingredients:</u>

- 3 egg whites
- 1/4 cup diced mushrooms
- 1/4 cup diced spinach
- 2 tablespoons diced onions
- Salt and pepper to taste

<u>Preparation:</u>

1. Whisk egg whites and pour them into a hot, non-stick skillet.

2. Add vegetables, season, and fold for a light and fluffy omelet.

These breakfast delights are not just easy on your kidneys but also a treat for your taste buds. Customize to your liking, and start your day on a delicious note. Here's to breakfast joy and the beginning of a flavorful day!A. Low-Potassium Breakfast Burrito

Cinnamon Oatmeal with Fresh Berries

If your mornings need a touch of warmth and a burst of fruity freshness, look no further! This Cinnamon Oatmeal with Fresh Berries is not just a breakfast; it's a melody that plays on your taste buds, setting the perfect tone for the day.

Ingredients:

- 1/2 cup old-fashioned oats
- 1 cup water or low-potassium milk
- 1/2 teaspoon ground cinnamon
- 1/4 cup fresh berries (blueberries, strawberries)

Preparation:

1. Cook the Oats

- In a saucepan, bring water or low-potassium milk to a gentle boil.
- Stir in the old-fashioned oats, and let them simmer over medium heat. Keep stirring occasionally to prevent sticking.

2. Add the Cinnamon Magic

- Once the oats begin to thicken, sprinkle in the enchanting ground cinnamon. Stir gently to infuse that warm, comforting aroma into every spoonful.

3. Berries on Top

- As the oats reach your desired consistency, turn off the heat.
- Spoon the cinnamon-kissed oatmeal into a bowl, and crown it with a vibrant medley of fresh berries. Let the colors dance together.

4. A Final Stir and Savor

- Gently mix the berries into the oatmeal, creating a delightful mosaic of textures and flavors.
- Take a moment to appreciate the symphony of warmth, sweetness, and freshness before taking your first blissful spoonful.

This Cinnamon Oatmeal with Fresh Berries is not just a breakfast; it's a celebration of simplicity and nourishment. The oats provide a comforting base, the cinnamon adds a touch of spice, and the fresh berries contribute a burst of natural sweetness. It's a morning melody that awakens your senses and sets the stage for a delightful day ahead. Here's to breakfast joy and the simple pleasures of a delicious start!

Lunch and Dinner Entrees

Lunch Delight:
Grilled Chicken Caesar Salad

Ingredients:
- Boneless, skinless chicken breasts
- Romaine lettuce
- Cherry tomatoes
- Parmesan cheese
- Caesar dressing
- Croutons

Preparation:
1. Marinate chicken in olive oil, garlic, and lemon juice.
2. Grill until perfectly charred and juicy.
3. Toss crisp romaine lettuce, halved cherry tomatoes, and shredded Parmesan.

4. Slice grilled chicken and place on the salad.

5. Drizzle with Caesar dressing, add croutons for crunch.

6. A flavorful lunch in under 30 minutes!

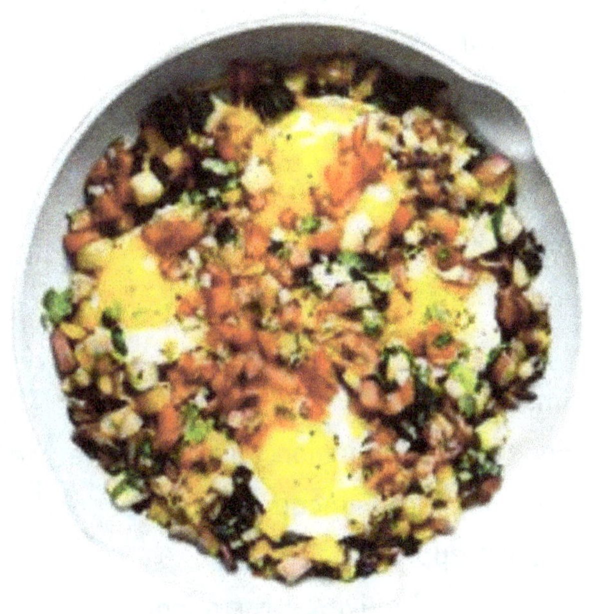

Pg31

Dinner Extravaganza:
<u>**Baked Salmon with Lemon Dill Sauce**</u>

Ingredients:
- Fresh salmon fillets
- Lemon
- Fresh dill
- Garlic
- Olive oil
- Salt and pepper

Preparation:
1. Preheat the oven and lay salmon on a baking sheet.
2. Squeeze fresh lemon juice over the filets.
3. Season with minced garlic, chopped dill, salt, and pepper.
4. Drizzle with olive oil for a moist finish.
5. Bake until salmon flakes easily with a fork.
6. Serve with a zesty lemon dill sauce on the side.
7. A sophisticated dinner that's both easy and elegant.

Grilled Lemon Herb Chicken

Grilled Lemon Herb Chicken Bliss

Ingredients:
- Chicken breasts
- Fresh lemons
- Olive oil
- Garlic cloves
- Fresh rosemary
- Thyme leaves
- Salt and pepper

Preparation:
1. Marinate chicken in a blend of olive oil, lemon juice, minced garlic, rosemary, thyme, salt, and pepper.
2. Allow it to soak up the flavors for at least 30 minutes.
3. Preheat the grill to medium-high heat.

4. Grill chicken until beautifully charred and fully cooked, ensuring juiciness.

5. Squeeze fresh lemon over the grilled perfection just before serving.

6. Garnish with chopped herbs for an extra burst of flavor.

7. A symphony of citrus and herbs that transforms a simple grilled dish into a culinary masterpiece.

Salmon with Dill Sauce

Succulent Salmon with Dill Sauce Elegance

Ingredients:
- Fresh salmon filets
- Fresh dill
- Greek yogurt
- Dijon mustard
- Lemon
- Garlic
- Salt and pepper

Preparation:
1. Lay salmon fillets on a baking sheet.
2. Mix Greek yogurt, finely chopped dill, Dijon mustard, minced garlic, and a squeeze of lemon for the sauce.
3. Season salmon with salt and pepper.

4. Spread a generous layer of the dill sauce over the filets.

5. Bake until the salmon flakes easily with a fork.

6. Garnish with additional fresh dill and a lemon wedge.

7. The harmony of creamy dill sauce and perfectly baked salmon a culinary symphony on your plate.

Enjoy this dish that effortlessly marries the richness of salmon with the refreshing zing of dill sauce, creating a delightful culinary experience for your taste buds!

Lentil and Vegetable Stew

Hearty Lentil and Vegetable Stew Comfort

Ingredients:
- Green or brown lentils
- Carrots
- Celery
- Onion
- Garlic
- Tomatoes
- Vegetable broth
- Bay leaves
- Cumin
- Paprika
- Salt and pepper
- Fresh parsley (for garnish)

Preparation:

1. Sauté diced onions and minced garlic in olive oil until fragrant.
2. Add chopped carrots and celery, cooking until slightly softened.
3. Stir in lentils, diced tomatoes, bay leaves, cumin, paprika, salt, and pepper.
4. Pour in vegetable broth, bringing the stew to a gentle boil.
5. Simmer until lentils are tender and flavors meld together.
6. Garnish with freshly chopped parsley before serving.
7. A warm bowl of nourishing lentil and vegetable stew—cozy, flavorful, and perfect for any season.

Delight in the heartiness of this stew, where wholesome lentils and vibrant vegetables come together in a symphony of flavors that will warm your soul with each comforting spoonful.

Snacks and Appetizers

Mouthwatering Caprese Skewers: A Bite-sized Delight

Ingredients:
- Fresh cherry tomatoes
- Fresh mozzarella balls
- Basil leaves
- Balsamic glaze
- Extra virgin olive oil
- Salt and pepper

Preparation:
1. Thread a cherry tomato, a folded basil leaf, and a mozzarella ball onto small skewers.
2. Arrange the skewers on a serving platter.
3. Drizzle with a mixture of balsamic glaze and extra virgin olive oil.
4. Sprinkle with a pinch of salt and a dash of pepper.

5. These caprese skewers offer a burst of freshness in every delightful bite.

Crispy Parmesan Zucchini Fries:
<u>**A Crunchy Sensation**</u>

Ingredients:
- Zucchini
- Panko breadcrumbs
- Grated Parmesan cheese
- Garlic powder
- Paprika
- Egg
- Marinara sauce (for dipping)

Preparation:
1. Cut zucchini into fry-shaped sticks.
2. Dip zucchini sticks in beaten egg, then coat with a mixture of Panko breadcrumbs, Parmesan, garlic powder, and paprika.
3. Bake until golden brown and crispy.
4. Serve with marinara sauce for a zesty kick.

5. A guilt-free indulgence that brings a satisfying crunch to your snack game.

Whether you're craving a fresh burst of flavors with Caprese Skewers or a crispy sensation with Parmesan Zucchini Fries, these snacks and appetizers are sure to elevate your taste buds to new heights.

Avocado and Tomato Salsa

Avocado and Tomato Salsa:
<u>A Zesty Dance of Flavors</u>

Ingredients:
- Ripe avocados
- Fresh tomatoes
- Red onion
- Jalapeño
- Fresh cilantro
- Lime
- Salt and pepper

Preparation:
1. Dice ripe avocados and tomatoes into bite-sized pieces.
2. Finely chop red onion, jalapeño (seeds removed for milder flavor), and fresh cilantro.
3. Combine all ingredients in a bowl.

4. Squeeze fresh lime juice over the mixture.

5. Gently toss and season with salt and pepper to taste.

6. Allow the flavors to meld for a few minutes.

7. Dive into the zesty goodness with tortilla chips or as a vibrant topping for your favorite dishes.

Indulge in the symphony of textures and tastes as creamy avocados and juicy tomatoes unite in this refreshing salsa. Perfect for dipping or as a lively accompaniment to your meals, it's a culinary celebration that dances on your palate.

Hummus with Crudites

**Savory Hummus with Vibrant Crudites:
A Garden Feast**

Ingredients:
- Chickpeas (canned or cooked)
- Tahini
- Garlic cloves
- Lemon
- Olive oil
- Cumin
- Paprika
- Salt
- Assorted fresh vegetables (carrots, cucumber, bell peppers, cherry tomatoes)

Preparation:
1. In a food processor, blend chickpeas, tahini, minced garlic, lemon juice, olive oil, cumin, paprika, and salt until smooth.
2. Adjust consistency with water if needed.
3. Transfer the hummus to a serving bowl.

4. Prepare a colorful array of fresh vegetables for dipping.
5. Dive into the creamy goodness of hummus paired with crisp, vibrant crudites.
6. A garden-inspired feast that's not only delicious but also a visual delight.

Elevate your snack experience with this delectable combination of velvety hummus and a rainbow of crunchy crudites. It's a celebration of flavors and textures that promises to bring joy to your taste buds.

Roasted Chickpeas

Roasted Chickpeas:
Crunchy Bites of Flavor Explosion

Ingredients:
- Canned chickpeas (drained and rinsed)
- Olive oil
- Smoked paprika
- Cumin
- Garlic powder
- Cayenne pepper (optional for a kick)
- Salt

Preparation:
1. Preheat the oven and pat chickpeas dry with a paper towel.
2. In a bowl, toss chickpeas with olive oil, smoked paprika, cumin, garlic powder, cayenne pepper, and a pinch of salt.
3. Spread the seasoned chickpeas on a baking sheet in a single layer.

4. Roast until golden and crispy, shaking the pan occasionally for even cooking.
5. Let them cool for a few minutes before indulging in the addictive crunch.
6. A healthy, protein-packed snack that's both satisfying and irresistibly flavorful.

Transform ordinary chickpeas into a crunchy delight with a burst of smoky, spicy, and savory flavors. Roasted to perfection, these little power-packed bites are the ultimate snack to elevate your munching experience.

Chapter 2: Desserts

Divine Chocolate Raspberry Tart:
A Symphony of Sweetness

Ingredients:
- Chocolate cookie crust
- Dark chocolate (for ganache)
- Fresh raspberries
- Heavy cream
- Sugar
- Vanilla extract

Preparation:
1. Melt dark chocolate and combine with warm heavy cream to create a velvety ganache.
2. Pour the ganache into a chocolate cookie crust, spreading it evenly.
3. Arrange fresh raspberries on top in a mesmerizing pattern.
4. Whip together heavy cream, sugar, and vanilla extract until soft peaks form.

5. Dollop the whipped cream on the tart for a cloud-like finish.

6. Chill the tart for a few hours to let the flavors meld.

7. Slice into this decadent creation—a luscious blend of rich chocolate and vibrant raspberries.

Indulge your sweet tooth with this exquisite Chocolate Raspberry Tart. Each bite is a harmonious dance of smooth chocolate, juicy raspberries, and airy whipped cream—a dessert that's not just a treat for the taste buds but a feast for the eyes.

Berry Parfait with Greek Yogurt

Berry Parfait with Greek Yogurt:
<u>Layers of Delight</u>

Ingredients:
- Mixed berries (strawberries, blueberries, raspberries)
- Greek yogurt
- Honey
- Granola
- Mint leaves (for garnish)

Preparation:
1. In a glass or bowl, layer Greek yogurt at the bottom for a creamy base.
2. Add a handful of mixed berries on top for a burst of freshness.
3. Drizzle honey over the berries, creating a sweet and tangy harmony.
4. Sprinkle a layer of granola for a satisfying crunch.

5. Repeat the layers until your parfait reaches the brim.

6. Finish with a dollop of Greek yogurt, a few berries, and a sprig of mint.

7. Dive into this delightful Berry Parfait, a wholesome treat that's as pleasing to the eyes as it is to the palate.

Embark on a journey of flavors with this Berry Parfait. The creamy Greek yogurt, luscious berries, and crunchy granola come together in perfect synergy, creating a visually appealing and irresistibly tasty dessert that's both simple and sophisticated.

Baked Apple with Cinnamon

**Baked Apple with Cinnamon:
<u>A Cozy Culinary Embrace</u>**

Ingredients:
- Apples (choose a variety like Honeycrisp or
Granny Smith)
- Cinnamon
- Brown sugar
- Butter
- Lemon juice
- Walnuts (optional, for topping)
- Vanilla ice cream (optional, for serving)

Preparation:
1. Preheat the oven and core the apples,
leaving the bottoms intact.
2. Mix cinnamon, brown sugar, and a touch of
melted butter in a bowl.
3. Stuff the apples with this sweet mixture.

4. Sprinkle a bit of lemon juice to enhance the natural flavors.
5. Bake until the apples are tender and aromatic.
6. Optionally, top with chopped walnuts for a delightful crunch.
7. Serve warm, perhaps with a scoop of vanilla ice cream for the ultimate indulgence.

Experience the magic of simplicity with Baked Apples infused with the warmth of cinnamon. This comforting dessert not only fills your home with a heavenly aroma but also promises a cozy, flavorful embrace that captures the essence of comfort and sweetness.

Beverages

Zesty Mint Lemonade:
<u>A Refreshing Citrus Symphony</u>

Ingredients:
- Fresh lemons
- Mint leaves
- Sugar
- Water
- Ice cubes

Preparation:
1. Squeeze the juice from fresh lemons into a pitcher.
2. In a separate container, make a mint-infused simple syrup by dissolving sugar in hot water and adding fresh mint leaves.
3. Strain the mint leaves and pour the syrup into the lemon juice.

4. Add cold water and stir until well combined.
5. Adjust sweetness to your liking by adding more sugar if needed.
6. Chill the lemonade for a couple of hours.
7. Serve over ice, garnished with mint leaves for a burst of freshness.

Quench your thirst with this Zesty Mint Lemonade— a harmonious blend of tangy lemons and cool mint that will transport you to a refreshing oasis. Perfect for warm days or any time you need a revitalizing sip of citrusy delight.

Hydration Tips for Kidney Health

Stay Sip-Happy with Citrus-Infused Water:

<u>Ingredients</u>: Water, sliced citrus fruits (lemons, limes, oranges)

<u>Preparation</u>: Infuse your water with citrus slices for a flavorful twist that not only enhances the taste but also provides a dose of kidney-loving antioxidants.

Cool as a Cucumber Hydration:

<u>Ingredients</u>: Water, cucumber slices

<u>Preparation</u>: Add cucumber slices to your water for a hydrating and refreshing beverage. Cucumbers are hydrating and low in potassium, making them kidney-friendly.

Berry-licious Antioxidant Boost:

Ingredients: Water, mixed berries (blueberries, strawberries)

Preparation: Berries are rich in antioxidants. Toss a handful into your water for a tasty and kidney-healthy hydration option.

Herbal Infusion Elixir:

Ingredients: Water, herbal teas (like mint or hibiscus)

Preparation: Brew a kidney-friendly herbal tea, cool it down, and enjoy a flavorful, caffeine-free option that contributes to your daily fluid intake.

Limit Sugary and Caffeinated Drinks:

Preparation: Reduce the intake of sugary and caffeinated beverages, as they can contribute to dehydration. Opt for water and kidney-friendly herbal teas instead.

Consult with a Dietitian:

<u>Preparation:</u> Work with a registered dietitian to tailor your hydration plan to your specific kidney health needs, considering factors like fluid restrictions and dietary requirements.

Maintaining proper hydration is crucial for kidney health. Incorporate these flavorful and kidney-friendly hydration tips into your routine to nourish your body's essential filters and support overall well-being.

Herbal Tea Infusions

Herbal Tea Infusions:
<u>Sip Your Way to Serenity</u>

Chamomile and Lavender Soothe-Tea:
<u>Ingredients:</u> Chamomile flowers, lavender buds
<u>Preparation:</u> Steep chamomile flowers and lavender buds in hot water for a calming blend that helps relax the mind and body.

Peppermint Passion Refresher:
<u>Ingredients:</u> Peppermint leaves
<u>Preparation:</u> Brew peppermint leaves for an invigorating and digestive-friendly infusion, perfect for a midday pick-me-up.

Lemon Ginger Zest Infusion:
<u>Ingredients:</u> Fresh ginger, lemon slices
<u>Preparation:</u> Combine fresh ginger slices and lemon in hot water for a zesty,

immune-boosting tea that adds a kick to your day.

Hibiscus Berry Bliss Brew:
<u>Ingredients:</u> Hibiscus petals, mixed berries
<u>Preparation:</u> Steep hibiscus petals and mixed berries for a vibrant and antioxidant-rich infusion that delights the senses.

Lemongrass Serenade Elixir:
<u>Ingredients:</u> Lemongrass stalks
<u>Preparation:</u> Infuse lemongrass stalks in hot water for a fragrant and citrusy tea that promotes relaxation and tranquility.

Rosemary Mint Revival Tonic:
<u>Ingredients:</u> Fresh rosemary, mint leaves
<u>Preparation:</u> Combine fresh rosemary and mint leaves in hot water for a revitalizing infusion that uplifts the spirit.

Embark on a journey of flavors with these herbal tea infusions. From the soothing Chamomile and Lavender Soothe-Tea to the invigorating Peppermint Passion Refresher, each sip is a delightful experience that brings both comfort and vitality to your day.

Fruit-Infused Water Recipes

Fruit-Infused Water Recipes:
<u>Quench Your Thirst with Nature's Sweetness</u>

Citrus Burst Bliss:
<u>Ingredients:</u> Water, sliced oranges, lemons, and limes
<u>Preparation:</u> Combine slices of oranges, lemons, and limes with water for a zesty and refreshing infusion that hydrates and invigorates.

Berry-Mint Fiesta Fusion:
<u>Ingredients:</u> Water, mixed berries (strawberries, blueberries, raspberries), fresh mint leaves
<u>Preparation:</u> Infuse water with a medley of berries and fresh mint leaves for a burst of antioxidants and a hint of minty coolness.

Cucumber Melon Oasis Refresher:

<u>Ingredients:</u> Water, cucumber slices, watermelon cubes

<u>Preparation:</u> Add crisp cucumber slices and juicy watermelon cubes to water for a hydrating and subtly sweet infusion that screams summer.

Tropical Pineapple Paradise Elixir:

<u>Ingredients:</u> Water, pineapple chunks, coconut water

<u>Preparation:</u> Combine pineapple chunks with water and a splash of coconut water for a tropical escape that's both hydrating and delicious.

Mango Ginger Zing Quencher:

<u>Ingredients:</u> Water, mango chunks, fresh ginger slices

<u>Preparation:</u> Infuse water with the sweetness of mango chunks and the zing of fresh ginger for a rejuvenating and flavorful beverage.

Herbal Citrus Infusion:

Ingredients: Water, basil leaves, citrus slices (orange, lemon)

Preparation: Elevate your water with the aromatic essence of basil leaves and slices of orange and lemon for a sophisticated herbal citrus infusion.

Transform your hydration routine with these delightful fruit-infused water recipes. Each sip is a journey through vibrant flavors, offering a delicious way to stay refreshed and nourished throughout the day.

Conclusion

Congratulations on completing your journey through this Renal Diet Cookbook for the newly diagnosed. As you turn the final page, remember that this isn't just a collection of recipes; it's a guide to nourishing your body, supporting your kidneys, and embracing a lifestyle that promotes well-being.

In these pages, you've discovered a symphony of ingredients carefully curated to align with renal health. From vibrant salads to comforting stews, each recipe is not just a delightful meal but a step towards better health. By understanding the significance of nutrient balance, portion control, and mindful choices, you've empowered yourself with the knowledge to make informed decisions about what goes on your plate.

This cookbook is a testament to the idea that a renal diet doesn't mean sacrificing flavor or variety. It's an opportunity to explore new tastes, experiment with wholesome ingredients, and savor the joy that a well-balanced diet brings. Through the richness of these recipes, you've embarked on a culinary journey that celebrates life, health, and the joy of good food.

As you navigate your newfound path, remember that this isn't a restrictive diet; it's a celebration of the incredible array of foods that contribute to your overall wellness. Use these recipes as a foundation, and don't be afraid to get creative in the kitchen. Let your taste buds guide you, and find joy in the process of discovering what truly nourishes and delights you.

Most importantly, remember that your journey to better renal health is unique. It's about finding what works best for you, listening to your body, and embracing a lifestyle that promotes not just physical health but also a sense of fulfillment and happiness.

May these recipes serve as a constant companion on your path to wellness. Here's to good health, delicious meals, and the fulfilling journey that lies ahead. Cheers to you and the vibrant, flavorful life you're creating!

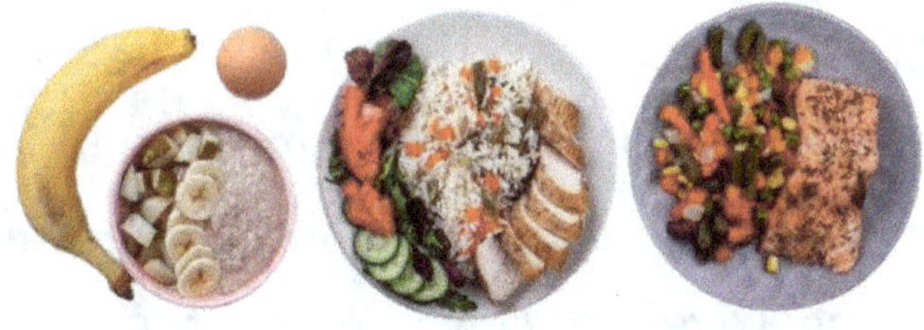

Dear Valued Reader,

I hope you enjoyed my book. I poured my heart and soul into it, and I'm so grateful that you took the time to read it.

If you found the book helpful, insightful, or entertaining, I would be honored if you would consider leaving a positive review. Your feedback means the world to me as an author, and it can help other potential readers discover my work.

Also, if you think there's are certain contents in the book which you don't really understand,or you have a suggestion towards this book please kindly send me a direct mail here

>>>>coachsolomon2@gmail.com<<<<

I will happy to help and respond happily

Thank you for your support!

You can also check out some of my compelling and interesting Biographies out on Amazon

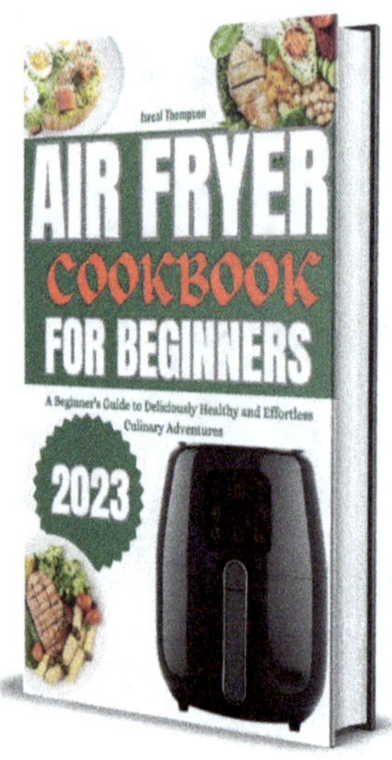

Copy and paste the link below on your browser to check it out

>>>>> https://a.co/d/4nrKaWl <<<<<

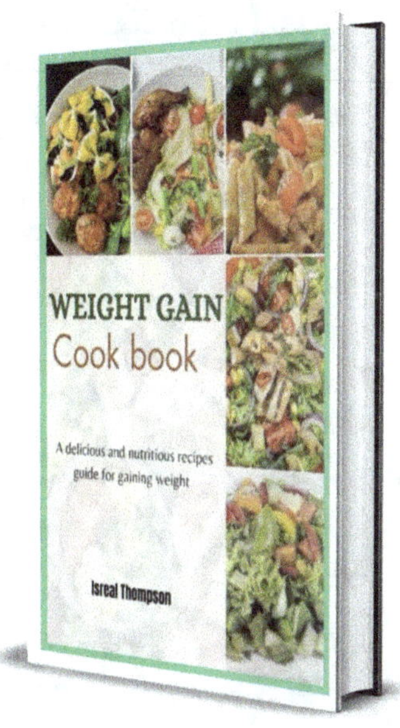

Copy and paste the link below on your browser to check it out

>>>> **https://a.co/d/bSGdGba** <<<<

Enjoy your renal recipes Adventures

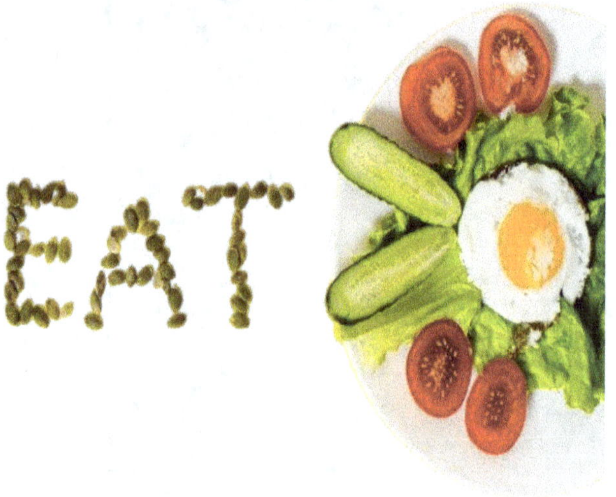